NIPAH VIRUS

Emerging Threats, Hidden Horizons Unveiled: and Understanding the Deadly Enigma"

By

Dr Buford. L. Brown

Table of contents

Introduction

In the realm of infectious diseases, where the invisible forces of nature can wreak havoc on human populations, few adversaries have emerged as enigmatic and menacing as the Nipah virus. Like a malevolent specter, it has haunted the annals of medical history, striking fear into the hearts of scientists, healthcare professionals, and the general public alike. Its tale is one of mystery, devastation, and relentless scientific pursuit, and it unfolds within the pages of this meticulously crafted tome, titled "NIPAH Virus."

This compelling opus is not just another book; it is a comprehensive exploration into the very heart of a viral threat that transcends geographical borders and human comprehension. From its shadowy origins deep within the rainforests of Southeast Asia to its ominous emergence as a global health concern, the Nipah virus stands as a stark reminder of the ever-present danger posed by zoonotic diseases.

In the corridors of science, where curiosity drives exploration and knowledge serves as both shield and sword, this book ventures boldly. It offers readers an unprecedented journey through the intricate labyrinth of Nipah virus research, taking them by the hand and leading them into the depths of this viral enigma. This is a narrative that traverses the boundaries of disciplines – virology, epidemiology, immunology, and more – in its quest for understanding, prevention, and ultimately, control.

The pages within are laden with stories of courage and sacrifice, of tireless individuals who have dedicated their lives to combating this insidious pathogen. It delves into the heroic efforts of healthcare workers who risk their lives on the frontlines, the tireless labor of researchers who toil in laboratories to unlock its secrets, and the solidarity of global communities uniting against a common enemy.

As you embark on this intellectual odyssey through the world of Nipah virus, prepare to be captivated by the narrative. From the virus's intricate structure and transmission dynamics to the profound human toll it exacts, each chapter unfolds like a gripping thriller. This book is an unwavering testament to the resilience of the human spirit in the face of adversity, a celebration of human ingenuity, and a stark reminder that our battles against microbial foes are not only in the realm of science but also in the arena of ethics, social responsibility, and global cooperation.

"NIPAH Virus" is not merely a book; it is a monument to the relentless pursuit of knowledge, a beacon of hope in the darkest of times, and a chronicle of humanity's unwavering determination to overcome the deadliest of foes. Prepare to be enlightened, engaged, and ultimately inspired, for within these pages, the Nipah virus, once shrouded in mystery and terror, is unveiled in all its complex, chilling glory.

Book Description

In the darkest corners of our world, unseen and unfelt until it strikes, lies a silent menace - the Nipah Virus. This insidious pathogen, known for its devastating impact, has sparked fear and intrigue across the globe. In the pages of "NIPAH Virus Unveiled: Understanding the Deadly Enigma," embark on a journey into the heart of this enigmatic disease, where science meets human drama in a gripping tale of survival, resilience, and the relentless pursuit of knowledge.

 Unveiling the Nipah Virus:

Delve deep into the microscopic world of virology as you discover the origins, structure, and behavior of the Nipah Virus. From its emergence in Malaysia to sporadic outbreaks in South Asia, this book traces the virus's chilling journey through history.

Effects on Human Health:

Experience the heart-wrenching stories of those who have faced the Nipah Virus head-on. Witness the physical and emotional toll it takes on its victims and their loved ones. Learn about the various strains and mutations, each with its unique set of symptoms and challenges.

Questions to Ponder:

As you turn each page, thought-provoking questions will fill your mind:

- What are the underlying causes of Nipah Virus outbreaks?
- How do we prevent and control the spread of this deadly disease?
- What are the current advancements in research and treatment?
- What is the global impact of Nipah Virus on healthcare systems and economies?

The Book's Promise:

This comprehensive guide equips you with a thorough understanding of the Nipah Virus, offering insights into the latest research, treatments, and prevention strategies. It acts as a beacon of hope for those who seek answers to questions that have long haunted the scientific community.

How This Book Can Help:

- Empower yourself with knowledge: Gain a deep understanding of the virus's biology, epidemiology, and prevention measures.
- Navigate the complexities: This book breaks down complex scientific concepts into easily digestible information, making it accessible to readers of all backgrounds.

- Stay informed: Stay up-to-date with the latest breakthroughs and findings related to Nipah Virus research.

Whether you're a concerned citizen, a healthcare professional, or a researcher, "NIPAH Virus Unveiled" offers a comprehensive and insightful exploration of this relentless adversary. By the time you turn the final page, you'll be armed with the knowledge needed to confront the Nipah Virus and champion the fight against this deadly enigma.

Don't wait in the shadows of ignorance. Join us on this enlightening journey into the world of Nipah Virus, where understanding is the key to survival. Grab your copy today and become part of the solution!

Chapter One

Introduction to Nipah Virus: A Lethal Threat

In the annals of infectious diseases, there exists a class of pathogens that captivate the imagination with their lethal potential, a group of viruses that stand as harbingers of doom for both humans and animals alike. Among this chilling pantheon of microbial villains, one insidious entity has emerged as a particularly menacing adversary: the Nipah virus. This nefarious pathogen, which belongs to the Paramyxoviridae family, Henipavirus genus, has garnered worldwide attention for its deadly outbreaks and capacity to spark fear in even the most seasoned epidemiologists.

Nipah virus, named after the village of Sungai Nipah in Malaysia where it was first identified in 1999, presents a multifaceted and elusive threat that continues to baffle scientists and healthcare professionals alike. Its complex biology, devastating clinical manifestations, and the potential for rapid spread have propelled it into the forefront of global health concerns.

This introductory exploration seeks to delve deep into the world of the Nipah virus, offering a comprehensive overview of its origins, structure, modes of transmission, clinical presentation, historical outbreaks, and the relentless quest for effective prevention and treatment strategies. By the time we conclude this journey, you will have gained a profound understanding of this enigmatic virus and the imperative need to address it as a global health priority.

The Origins of Nipah Virus

Nipah virus made its ominous debut in the small village of Sungai Nipah, Malaysia, in 1999, when a cluster of severe encephalitis cases emerged among pig farmers and their families. This perplexing outbreak initially stumped medical experts, but diligent investigation eventually unveiled the virus responsible for the tragedy. The fruit bats of the Pteropus genus were identified as the natural reservoir of the virus, shedding light on the complex interplay between wildlife and emerging diseases.

The Viral Architecture

At the heart of understanding the Nipah virus lies a grasp of its intricate structure. This enveloped, single-stranded RNA virus possesses a unique fusion protein (F) that facilitates its entry into host cells, and a glycoprotein (G) that interacts with host receptors, enabling cell attachment. This architectural complexity contributes to its ability to invade the central nervous system, a key factor in its deadly pathogenesis.

Modes of Transmission

Nipah virus is not only an enigma in terms of its origin and structure but also in the diverse ways it can be transmitted. While direct contact with infected bats or their secretions is a known risk, human-to-human transmission has been a recurring nightmare during outbreaks. Pigs, acting as intermediate hosts, can amplify and spread the virus, highlighting the intricate web of potential vectors.

Clinical Presentation

The clinical presentation of Nipah virus infection is nothing short of terrifying. Initial symptoms often mimic those of common respiratory illnesses, making early diagnosis a daunting challenge. However, as the virus progresses, it can cause severe encephalitis, characterized by seizures, altered mental status, and a mortality rate that can surpass 70% in some outbreaks. This lethal blend of symptoms serves as a chilling reminder of Nipah's formidable reputation.

Historical Outbreaks

The global community has witnessed the ravaging impact of Nipah virus through several devastating outbreaks. From its inaugural emergence in Malaysia in 1999 to subsequent outbreaks in Bangladesh and India, each episode has left a trail of tragedy and despair in its wake. The unpredictability of these outbreaks and their potential to rapidly escalate into large-scale epidemics underscore the urgent need for effective control measures.

The Quest for Prevention and Treatment

In the face of this lethal menace, scientists, healthcare workers, and policymakers have tirelessly sought ways to prevent and treat Nipah virus infections. Research into vaccines and antiviral therapies has progressed, but challenges persist. Balancing the need for effective medical interventions with the conservation of bat populations, which serve crucial ecological roles, is a delicate and ongoing ethical dilemma.

As we embark on this journey through the labyrinthine world of Nipah virus, we must remember that this is not merely an exploration of a pathogen; it is a testament to the resilience and ingenuity of humanity in the face of a relentless adversary. The story of Nipah virus is one that bridges the realms of science, ecology, and public health, serving as a stark reminder that our planet's health is inextricably linked to our own.

Join us in this odyssey as we unravel the mysteries of Nipah virus, explore the global efforts to combat its menace, and ultimately confront the stark reality of a lethal threat that continues to cast a long shadow over our world.

Chapter Two

The Emergence of Nipah: From Bats to Humans

1: Prologue - A Mysterious Malady

In the quiet rural regions of Malaysia, nestled amongst lush greenery and dense forests, an invisible menace was about to reveal itself. It was 1998 when the Nipah virus, a hitherto unknown and deadly pathogen, first emerged, setting in motion a series of events that would forever change our understanding of zoonotic diseases and their transmission to humans.

2: Bats as Silent Carriers

At the heart of the Nipah virus's emergence lies the enigmatic world of bats. Bats, often regarded as nature's nocturnal aviators, have long been recognized as potential reservoirs for various viruses. These flying mammals, found in large colonies across Southeast Asia, play a pivotal role in the Nipah virus's life cycle, silently carrying and shedding the virus without displaying any signs of illness themselves.

3: Unveiling the Culprit - Fruit Bats

Within the vast realm of bat species, it was the fruit bats, specifically the Pteropus genus, that took center stage in the Nipah virus saga. Scientists traced the origins of the virus to these bats, particularly the Pteropus hypomelanus species. The bats' habit of foraging for fruits in orchards situated near human settlements provided the ideal opportunity for viral spillover.

4: Viral Spillover – Bridging the Gap

The Nipah virus's journey from bats to humans involves a complex interplay of ecological factors. This chapter delves into the intricate mechanisms that allow the virus to bridge the gap between its bat hosts and human victims, including the contamination of date palm sap, a delicacy consumed in the region.

5: The Human Toll – A Deadly Outbreak

The year 1998 marked the first recorded outbreak of Nipah virus in Malaysia. This chapter recounts the harrowing experiences of those affected, detailing the rapid and severe symptoms that befell the victims. The virus's ability to cause encephalitis and acute respiratory distress syndrome made it a formidable adversary, claiming numerous lives in its wake.

6: The Race Against Time - Scientific Investigations

As the Nipah virus wreaked havoc, a global race to understand and combat the virus began. This chapter highlights the tireless efforts of scientists and healthcare professionals who worked relentlessly to identify the virus, develop diagnostic tools, and implement control measures to contain the outbreak.

7: **Lessons from Malaysia - A Paradigm Shift**

The Malaysian outbreak served as a wake-up call for the scientific community and public health authorities worldwide. This chapter explores the paradigm shift in our approach to emerging infectious diseases, emphasizing the importance of surveillance, early detection, and rapid response.

8: **Beyond Malaysia - Global Implications**

Nipah virus, it turned out, was not confined to Malaysia alone. This chapter traces the virus's subsequent outbreaks in Bangladesh and India, underlining the global implications of this emerging pathogen. It also discusses the challenges of managing outbreaks in resource-constrained settings.

9: **From Virus to Vaccine - A Glimmer of Hope**

Despite the devastation caused by Nipah virus outbreaks, there is hope on the horizon. This chapter delves into the ongoing efforts to develop vaccines and therapeutics to protect both humans and animals from this deadly virus.

10: **Nipah Virus in the 21st Century - A Continuing Threat**

The final chapter brings us to the present day, where the Nipah virus continues to pose a significant threat. It discusses the ongoing research, preparedness measures, and the importance of coexisting with wildlife while minimising the risk of zoonotic spillover events.

Epilogue: The Ongoing Quest for Knowledge

The Nipah virus saga serves as a reminder of the intricate web of interactions that exist between humans, animals, and the environment. It underscores the need for continued vigilance, research, and global cooperation in our quest to understand and mitigate emerging infectious diseases.

Acknowledgments: A Tribute to Those Who Fought

This section pays homage to the countless individuals and organizations whose dedication, sacrifice, and collaborative efforts have contributed to our understanding of Nipah virus and our ability to respond to its threats.

Bibliography: A Deep Dive into Nipah Virus

For those who wish to explore the Nipah virus further, this comprehensive bibliography provides a curated list of scientific papers, books, and resources that delve into various aspects of this fascinating and deadly pathogen.

Index: Navigating the Nipah Virus Journey

A detailed index allows readers to easily locate specific topics, names, and events throughout the book, facilitating a deeper understanding of the Nipah virus's emergence and impact.

With "NIPAH Virus: The Emergence of a Deadly Pathogen - From Bats to Humans," we embark on a comprehensive exploration of a virus that has challenged our scientific understanding and reshaped our approach to emerging infectious diseases. This narrative seeks to inform, educate, and inspire future generations to continue the quest for knowledge and vigilance in the face of evolving threats from the natural world.

Chapter Three

Nipah Virus Outbreaks: A Global Perspective

The Nipah virus, a zoonotic pathogen, has garnered significant attention in recent years due to its potential for causing severe outbreaks with high mortality rates. This chapter provides an in-depth exploration of Nipah virus outbreaks on a global scale, shedding light on its history, transmission, epidemiology, and the challenges faced by healthcare systems in managing this deadly virus.

Historical Context

The Nipah virus was first identified in Malaysia in 1999 when it caused an outbreak among pig farmers and subsequently spread to humans, resulting in severe respiratory and neurological symptoms. The source of the virus was traced to fruit bats, which served as natural reservoirs. This incident marked the emergence of a new zoonotic virus with the potential to cause large-scale outbreaks.

Epidemiology

Geographical Distribution

Nipah virus outbreaks have primarily occurred in Southeast Asia, particularly in Malaysia, Bangladesh, and India. These regions have witnessed sporadic outbreaks over the years, with varying levels of severity. However, with globalization and increased human mobility, the virus has the potential to reach other parts of the world, making it a global health concern.

Transmission

Human infections typically occur through close contact with infected animals or consumption of contaminated food, such as date palm sap, which bats may have contaminated with their saliva or urine. Human-to-human transmission has also been documented, particularly in healthcare settings, raising concerns about the virus's pandemic potential.

Clinical Presentation

Nipah virus infection presents with a range of symptoms, including fever, headache, dizziness, and confusion. In severe cases, it can progress to encephalitis, characterized by seizures and altered consciousness. The case fatality rate varies but can be as high as 75%, making Nipah virus one of the deadliest zoonotic pathogens.

Challenges and Responses

Diagnosis

One of the key challenges in managing Nipah virus outbreaks is the timely and accurate diagnosis. Molecular tests like polymerase chain reaction (PCR) and serological assays are essential for confirming cases, but their availability and accessibility in affected regions can be limited.

Prevention and Control

Preventing Nipah virus outbreaks requires a multifaceted approach. This includes raising awareness among communities about safe food practices, reducing exposure to infected animals, and implementing strict infection control measures in healthcare settings. Developing a vaccine is another crucial step in preventing future outbreaks.

The Global Response

The World Health Organization (WHO) and other international agencies have been actively involved in responding to Nipah virus outbreaks. They provide technical support, facilitate research, and assist countries in strengthening their surveillance and response capabilities.

Chapter Four

Clinical Manifestations of Nipah Virus Infection

In the annals of infectious diseases, the Nipah virus (NiV) has emerged as a formidable and enigmatic pathogen, garnering global attention for its devastating clinical manifestations. This chapter delves into the intricate tapestry of clinical manifestations associated with Nipah virus infection, offering a comprehensive exploration of this pathogenic menace.

Historical Perspective:

1. To embark on this odyssey through the clinical manifestations of Nipah virus infection, it is essential to first understand the historical context. Nipah virus was first identified in 1998 during an outbreak in Malaysia, where it was responsible for a cluster of severe respiratory and neurological illnesses. Since then, NiV has continued to pose a substantial threat to public health, with sporadic outbreaks reported in various parts of Southeast Asia, including Bangladesh and India.

Transmission and Pathogenesis:

2. Nipah virus primarily spreads from bats to humans through intermediate hosts, such as pigs or date palm sap contaminated by bat excretions. The virus's ability to adapt and evolve has allowed it to cross species barriers, making it a dynamic and ever-evolving threat. Following transmission, NiV gains entry into the human body and begins its insidious journey, targeting multiple organ systems.

Incubation Period:

3. The incubation period for Nipah virus infection ranges from 4 to 14 days. During this period, infected individuals remain asymptomatic, which poses a significant challenge for early detection and containment.

4.

Clinical Spectrum

5. The clinical manifestations of Nipah virus infection are diverse and can be categorized into two broad syndromes: respiratory and encephalitic. The presentation of symptoms can vary widely, with some individuals remaining asymptomatic while others develop severe illness.

6. Respiratory Manifestations:

* Initially, patients may experience flu-like symptoms, including fever, cough, and sore throat.

* As the infection progresses, respiratory distress becomes pronounced, leading to acute respiratory distress syndrome (ARDS).

* Chest X-rays often reveal bilateral lung infiltrates, a hallmark of severe NiV infection.

6. Neurological Manifestations:

* Perhaps the most ominous aspect of Nipah virus infection is its propensity to cause encephalitis.

* Neurological symptoms include altered mental status, confusion, seizures, and focal neurological deficits.

* Magnetic resonance imaging (MRI) may show characteristic findings, such as bilateral thalamic lesions.

7. Gastrointestinal Symptoms:

* Nausea, vomiting, and abdominal pain are common gastrointestinal manifestations of NiV infection.

- Hepatitis can also occur, with elevated liver enzymes and jaundice observed in some cases.

8. Hematological Abnormalities:

- Nipah virus infection often leads to thrombocytopenia and lymphocytosis, contributing to bleeding tendencies and immune dysregulation.

9. Multi-Organ Dysfunction:

- As the disease progresses, multi-organ dysfunction syndrome (MODS) can ensue, involving the heart, kidneys, and liver.

- This cascade of organ failure further complicates the clinical picture and increases the risk of mortality.

10. Prognosis and Treatment:

- The mortality rate associated with Nipah virus infection varies, with reported case fatality rates ranging from 40% to 90%.

- Currently, there is no specific antiviral treatment for NiV infection, and management is largely supportive.

Chapter Five

Diagnosis and Laboratory Techniques

The diagnosis of infectious diseases has undergone a significant transformation in recent years, owing to advances in laboratory techniques and our understanding of various pathogens. The NPAH (New Pathogenic Animal-Human) virus, an emerging viral threat, demands a comprehensive and sophisticated approach to its diagnosis. This chapter delves into the various laboratory techniques and diagnostic methods employed in the identification and confirmation of NPAH virus infections. These techniques are essential for understanding the virus's epidemiology, tracking its spread, and developing effective intervention strategies.

I. Clinical Presentation:

Before discussing the laboratory techniques, it is crucial to understand the clinical presentation of NIPAH virus infections. Clinical signs and symptoms can be non-specific, making it challenging to distinguish NOAH from other similar diseases. Common clinical features include fever, respiratory distress, myalgia, and gastrointestinal symptoms. Severe cases may progress to acute respiratory distress syndrome (ARDS), multi-organ failure, and death. Clinical suspicion and epidemiological context often guide the decision to initiate laboratory testing.

II. Sample Collection:

Collecting appropriate specimens is the first step in diagnosing NIPAH virus infections. Respiratory specimens, such as nasopharyngeal swabs, throat swabs, or bronchoalveolar lavage, are the primary samples of choice due to the virus's respiratory route of transmission. Blood, urine, and stool samples may also be collected for further investigations.

III. Molecular Diagnostic Techniques:

1. Reverse Transcription Polymerase Chain Reaction (RT-PCR):

RT-PCR is the gold standard for NIPAH virus diagnosis. It detects viral RNA in clinical specimens. This technique offers high sensitivity and specificity, making it invaluable for early diagnosis and monitoring of viral load. Multiplex RT-PCR assays can simultaneously detect multiple respiratory viruses, aiding in differential diagnosis.

2. Next-Generation Sequencing (NGS):

NGS allows for the comprehensive analysis of viral genetic material. It can help identify viral subtypes, mutations, and trace transmission chains. Whole-genome sequencing using NGS provides valuable insights into the virus's evolution and adaptation to human hosts.

IV. Serological Testing:

Serological assays detect antibodies produced by the host in response to NPAH virus infection. Enzyme-linked immunosorbent assays (ELISAs) and neutralization assays are commonly used. Serology is crucial for identifying past infections, understanding seroprevalence in the population, and assessing immunity.

V. Viral Culture:

Viral culture involves growing the NPAH virus in cell culture systems. Although time-consuming and labor-intensive, it provides valuable information about viral replication dynamics and allows for the isolation of live virus for further research and vaccine development.

VI. Antigen Detection:

Immunofluorescence assays (IFA) and enzyme immunoassays (EIA) can detect viral antigens in clinical specimens. These tests are particularly useful for rapid diagnosis, but their sensitivity may vary.

VII. Point-of-Care Tests:

Point-of-care tests, such as rapid antigen tests and molecular assays, are becoming increasingly important for timely diagnosis, especially in resource-limited settings. These tests provide quick results and are crucial for containing outbreaks.

VIII. Radiological Imaging:

Chest X-rays and computed tomography (CT) scans can reveal characteristic lung abnormalities associated with NPAH virus infection, aiding in the clinical assessment and differential diagnosis.

IX. Laboratory Biosafety:

Handling specimens and conducting diagnostic tests for NPAH virus requires adherence to stringent biosafety protocols to prevent laboratory-acquired infections. Biosafety level 2 (BSL-2) and BSL-3 facilities are typically used, depending on the procedure.

Chapter Six

Nipah Virus Transmission and Prevention

In the realm of infectious diseases, few pathogens have evoked as much concern and intrigue as the Nipah virus. Emerging from the depths of the natural world, this virus has caused sporadic outbreaks with alarming mortality rates. The key to understanding and combating Nipah virus lies in comprehending its transmission dynamics and implementing robust prevention measures. In this chapter, we embark on an intricate journey through the intricate web of Nipah virus transmission pathways and explore the array of preventive strategies that have been devised to safeguard human and animal populations from its deadly grasp.

Nipah Virus: A Menace Emerges:

Nipah virus (NiV) is a member of the Paramyxoviridae family, a genus known as Henipavirus, and was first identified in Malaysia in 1998. Since then, it has made periodic appearances across Southeast Asia and South Asia, causing severe respiratory and neurological diseases in humans, as well as devastating outbreaks in animals. NiV is an enveloped, single-stranded RNA virus with a unique mode of transmission that poses significant challenges to containment and control.

Transmission Pathways:

Bat-to-Human Transmission:

1. The primary reservoir of Nipah virus is fruit bats of the Pteropodidae family. These bats, especially the Pteropus species, harbor the virus without showing clinical signs. Human infections often occur through the consumption of contaminated fruits or date palm sap, which have been contaminated by bat saliva, urine, or feces. Direct contact with infected bats or their bodily fluids can also lead to transmission.

Human-to-Human Transmission:

3. Once the virus enters the human population, it can be transmitted from person to person through respiratory secretions, including respiratory droplets and aerosols. This mode of transmission has been responsible for sustained outbreaks, particularly in healthcare settings, where close contact between infected patients and healthcare workers can facilitate transmission.

Animal-to-Human Transmission:

5. Nipah virus can infect a range of domestic animals, including pigs, dogs, and horses. Humans can become

infected when they come into contact with these infected animals, their tissues, or secretions. The amplification of the virus within pigs has been a significant contributor to large-scale outbreaks, as seen in Malaysia and Bangladesh.

Prevention Strategies:

Surveillance and Early Detection:

1. Early detection of Nipah virus outbreaks is critical for containment. Surveillance programs that monitor bat populations, animal health, and human cases enable rapid response efforts.

2.

3. Healthcare workers must use appropriate PPE, including masks, gloves, gowns, and eye protection when caring for Nipah virus-infected patients to minimize the risk of nosocomial transmission.

4.

Hygiene and Safe Practices:

5. Promoting good hygiene practices, such as handwashing and safe food handling, can reduce the risk of exposure to contaminated materials.

6.

Vaccination

7. Research into Nipah virus vaccines is ongoing, with promising candidates in development. Vaccination of

high-risk populations, such as healthcare workers and individuals in endemic areas, could play a crucial role in prevention.

Chapter Seven

Nipah Virus Treatment and Therapeutics

Nipah virus (NiV) is a zoonotic virus that belongs to the Paramyxoviridae family and was first identified in Malaysia in 1999 during an outbreak. Since then, it has emerged as a significant public health concern due to its high fatality rate and potential for human-to-human transmission. The absence of a specific antiviral drug or vaccine for Nipah virus has spurred intensive research efforts to develop effective treatments and therapeutics. This article delves into the latest advancements and strategies in Nipah virus treatment and therapeutics.

Understanding Nipah Virus:

Nipah virus is primarily transmitted to humans through direct contact with infected animals, such as fruit bats, or through consumption of contaminated fruits and raw date palm sap. It can also spread from person to person through respiratory secretions, making it highly contagious. Nipah virus infection can lead to severe respiratory and neurological symptoms, including encephalitis, making early intervention crucial.

Current Treatment Approaches:

As of my knowledge cutoff date in September 2021, there was no specific antiviral drug approved for the treatment of Nipah virus infection. Therefore, management mainly focused on supportive care, including mechanical ventilation and intensive care for severe cases. However, research was actively ongoing to identify potential therapeutic options.

Promising Antiviral Candidates:

Several antiviral candidates had shown promise in preclinical studies and were under evaluation for their effectiveness against Nipah virus. Some of these candidates included:

1. Ribavirin: Although not specifically designed for Nipah virus, ribavirin had shown some efficacy in vitro and in animal models. Clinical trials were being conducted to assess its effectiveness in humans.

2. Monoclonal Antibodies: Monoclonal antibodies were being developed to target the Nipah virus envelope glycoprotein. These antibodies had the potential to neutralize the virus and reduce disease severity.

3. RNA Interference (RNAi) Therapy: RNAi-based approaches were under investigation to inhibit Nipah virus replication at the genetic level. These therapies aimed to silence specific viral genes and halt viral propagation.

4. Viral Entry Inhibitors: Researchers were exploring compounds that could block the virus from entering human cells, preventing infection.

Vaccine Development:

Vaccine development for Nipah virus was another area of active research. Several vaccine candidates, including subunit vaccines and viral vector-based vaccines, were in various stages of development. These vaccines aimed to stimulate the immune system to produce protective antibodies against the virus.

Combination Therapies:

Combination therapies, involving a combination of antiviral drugs and immunomodulatory agents, were being investigated to enhance treatment outcomes and reduce the risk of drug resistance.

Challenges in Nipah Virus Treatment:

Developing effective treatments and therapeutics for Nipah virus posed several challenges:

1. Lack of Clinical Data: Limited clinical data and the rarity of Nipah virus outbreaks made it challenging to conduct robust clinical trials.

2. Animal Model Suitability: Finding appropriate animal models that accurately mimic human Nipah virus infection was a hurdle for preclinical testing.

3. Rapid Diagnosis: Early diagnosis of Nipah virus infection was crucial for effective treatment. Developing rapid diagnostic tests was a priority.

4. Global Preparedness: Nipah virus outbreaks primarily occurred in specific regions, making global preparedness and distribution of treatments and vaccines a logistical challenge.

Chapter Eight

Socioeconomic Impact and Public Health Responses

The Nipah virus (NiV) is a zoonotic virus that has garnered significant attention due to its severe public health implications. Since its discovery in 1999 in Malaysia, Nipah virus outbreaks have occurred sporadically in South and Southeast Asia, causing concern among global health organizations. This chapter delves into the multifaceted aspects of the socioeconomic impact of Nipah virus outbreaks and the subsequent public health responses that have been implemented to mitigate its consequences.

Socio Economic Impact:

1. Loss of Human Capital: Nipah virus outbreaks result in significant mortality rates, leading to the loss of valuable human resources within affected communities. The death toll among healthcare workers and caregivers can further exacerbate the shortage of skilled professionals.

2. Agricultural Disruptions: Due to its zoonotic nature, Nipah virus often originates from fruit bats and is transmitted to humans through intermediate hosts like pigs. Consequently, culling of pigs or suspension of pig

farming has a detrimental impact on the livelihoods of farmers and the agriculture industry.

3. Economic Decline: Affected regions often witness a downturn in economic activities. Fear of infection leads to reduced tourism, decreased consumer spending, and disruption of trade, thereby affecting local and regional economies.

4. Strain on Healthcare Systems: Nipah outbreaks strain healthcare systems, both financially and operationally. Hospitals and clinics become overwhelmed, diverting resources away from other essential medical services.

5. Stigmatization and Isolation: Communities impacted by Nipah outbreaks often face stigmatization, which can hinder social and economic recovery. People from affected regions may face discrimination, making it challenging to reintegrate into society.

Public Health Responses:

1. Surveillance and Early Detection: Effective surveillance systems are crucial for early detection of Nipah outbreaks. This includes monitoring both animal populations, particularly bats and pigs, and human cases. Timely identification allows for a rapid response.

2. Isolation and Quarantine: Infected individuals need to be isolated to prevent further transmission. Close contacts are quarantined, and healthcare workers are trained in infection prevention and control measures.

3. Vaccination and Treatment: Research into Nipah vaccines and treatments is ongoing. Developing effective medical countermeasures is a priority to reduce mortality rates.

4. Risk Communication: Effective risk communication is vital to dispel misinformation and reduce panic. Public health agencies need to engage with communities to ensure they understand the virus, its transmission, and protective measures.

5. One Health Approach: Recognizing the zoonotic origin of Nipah, a holistic "One Health" approach is crucial. This involves collaboration between human health, animal health, and environmental agencies to identify and mitigate risks at the animal-human interface.

6. Community Engagement: Engaging communities in outbreak response is essential. Local knowledge and practices can be integrated into control measures, and

community leaders can play a vital role in conveying public health messages.

Chapter Nine

Lessons from Nipah Virus: Preparedness for Future Pandemics

The Nipah virus outbreak that occurred in various parts of Asia in the late 1990s and early 2000s sent shockwaves through the global healthcare community. With its high mortality rate and capacity for human-to-human transmission, it served as a stark reminder of the potential for emerging infectious diseases to wreak havoc on societies unprepared for their arrival. As we stand on the precipice of a new era, marked by unprecedented global connectivity and the specter of ever-evolving pathogens, it is imperative that we learn from the lessons of Nipah virus and invest in preparedness for future pandemics.

Lesson 1: Early Detection and Surveillance:

One of the most critical lessons from the Nipah virus outbreak is the importance of early detection and surveillance. The delay in identifying the virus allowed it to spread unchecked, causing extensive damage before containment measures were put in place. Future pandemics can be mitigated through robust surveillance systems that track emerging diseases and provide real-time data to health authorities.

Lesson 2: International Collaboration:

The Nipah virus transcended borders, and it became clear that international collaboration is essential for pandemic preparedness. In our interconnected world, a disease outbreak in one corner can quickly become a global threat. Building stronger partnerships between nations, sharing information, and coordinating responses are pivotal to preventing and managing future pandemics.

Lesson 3: Research and Vaccine Development:

The development of vaccines and antiviral treatments for Nipah virus has been slow, but it highlights the need for accelerated research into emerging pathogens. Investing in research to understand these viruses and develop vaccines or treatments in advance is crucial. It not only saves lives but also prevents economic disruptions caused by extended lockdowns and restrictions.

Lesson 4: Public Health Infrastructure:

Nipah virus exposed the vulnerabilities in public health infrastructure in affected regions. Hospitals were overwhelmed, and healthcare workers faced significant risks. Investing in healthcare infrastructure, training healthcare workers, and ensuring adequate resources are available during pandemics is essential.

Lesson 5: Public Awareness and Education:

Misinformation and fear exacerbated the Nipah virus outbreak. Public awareness campaigns and education can be powerful tools in controlling the spread of infectious diseases. Governments and organizations must prioritize clear and accurate communication to keep the public informed and dispel rumors.

Lesson 6: One Health Approach:

Nipah virus, like many zoonotic diseases, originated in animals. Adopting a "One Health" approach that integrates human, animal, and environmental health is essential for preventing future pandemics. Surveillance of animal reservoirs, responsible wildlife management, and understanding the ecological factors contributing to disease transmission are vital components of this approach.

Chapter Ten

Beyond Nipah: Emerging Infectious Diseases and One Health Approach

Emerging infectious diseases (EIDs) pose a significant threat to global public health, economy, and social stability. Among these, Nipah virus, which was first identified in 1999 in Malaysia, stands as a harrowing example of the potential consequences of EIDs. The Nipah virus outbreak resulted in substantial mortality and economic losses, underscoring the urgent need for comprehensive strategies to combat such threats. The One Health approach is one such strategy that has gained prominence in recent years, offering a holistic framework to address the complex interplay between human, animal, and environmental health in the context of EIDs.

I. Nipah Virus: A Looming Menace

Historical Perspective:

> The Nipah virus is zoonotic in nature, with fruit bats acting as natural reservoirs. Its emergence in Malaysia in 1999, with subsequent outbreaks in India and Bangladesh, raised alarm bells within the global health community.

Clinical Manifestations:

2. Nipah virus infection in humans presents with a range of symptoms, from mild fever to severe encephalitis. The high mortality rate and lack of specific treatments make it a formidable threat.

Economic Impact:

3. Beyond the immediate health consequences, Nipah outbreaks result in substantial economic losses, primarily affecting agriculture and tourism industries.

II. The One Health Approach: A Comprehensive Paradigm

Defining One Health:

1. The One Health approach recognizes the interconnectedness of human, animal, and environmental health. It seeks to address health challenges at the interface of these domains.

2. Key Principles:

- Interdisciplinary collaboration
- Early detection and response
- Preventive measures
- Environmental stewardship

The Role of Surveillance:

3. Timely surveillance of potential zoonotic threats is crucial. It involves monitoring animal health, human cases, and environmental factors, such as habitat changes.

III. Nipah and the One Health Approach

Zoonotic Origins:

1. Nipah virus spillover events highlight the need for understanding and mitigating the factors that drive these cross-species transmissions.

Bat-Human Interface:

2. Research into the interactions between fruit bats and humans is essential to pinpoint risk factors and potential intervention points.

Agriculture and Livestock:

3. The One Health approach recognizes the role of livestock and agriculture in zoonotic disease transmission and emphasizes sustainable practices.

IV. The Global Response

International Collaboration:

1. Effective response to Nipah and other EIDs demands international cooperation and information sharing, transcending geopolitical boundaries.

Research and Innovation:

2. Ongoing research is vital for developing diagnostics, therapeutics, and vaccines to combat Nipah and other emerging threats.

V. Beyond Nipah: The Ongoing Challenge

EID Preparedness:

1. Nipah serves as a reminder of the unpredictable nature of EIDs. Global preparedness measures, including stockpiling medical supplies and building healthcare infrastructure, are imperative.

Climate Change and EIDs:

2. Environmental changes, driven by climate change, can alter the distribution of vector-borne diseases, including Nipah, necessitating adaptive strategies.

Conclusion

The NPah virus, with its complex and intriguing characteristics, presents a formidable challenge in the realm of virology and public health. As we delve deeper into the intricacies of this enigmatic pathogen, we are confronted with a multifaceted tapestry of factors that demand our attention and understanding. From its elusive origins to its potential for rapid mutation, the NPah virus emerges as a resilient adversary in the ongoing battle against infectious diseases.

One of the most striking aspects of the NPah virus is its ability to adapt and evolve. Its high mutation rate, combined with its zoonotic potential, poses a perpetual threat to human and animal populations alike. This adaptability underscores the importance of continuous surveillance and research to stay one step ahead of this ever-changing foe. In doing so, we can hope to develop effective diagnostic tools and therapeutic interventions that can mitigate the impact of the virus on global health.

Furthermore, the NPah virus serves as a poignant reminder of the interconnectedness of our world. As international travel and trade facilitate the movement of people and goods across borders, so too can infectious agents traverse continents with ease. This underscores the imperative for global cooperation in monitoring and responding to emerging infectious diseases, where timely information sharing and coordinated efforts can make all the difference in preventing widespread outbreaks.

The study of the NPah virus also reveals the incredible complexity of the host-pathogen interaction. Its ability to manipulate the host's immune system and evade detection is a testament to the sophisticated strategies that viruses employ for survival. Unraveling these intricate mechanisms not only enhances our understanding of virology but also provides insights into potential therapeutic targets for future antiviral drug development.

In conclusion, the NPah virus stands as a formidable challenge on the frontlines of infectious disease research. Its adaptability, zoonotic potential, and global reach demand our unwavering attention and collaborative efforts. As we continue to delve into the mysteries of this virus, we are not only advancing our knowledge of virology but also working towards a safer and healthier future for humanity. It is through our collective dedication to science and public health that we can hope to triumph over this enigmatic adversary and secure a brighter tomorrow.